School Based & Pediatric Occupational Therapy Resource Series:

Quick Pediatric Fine Motor and Sensory Screener and Assessment

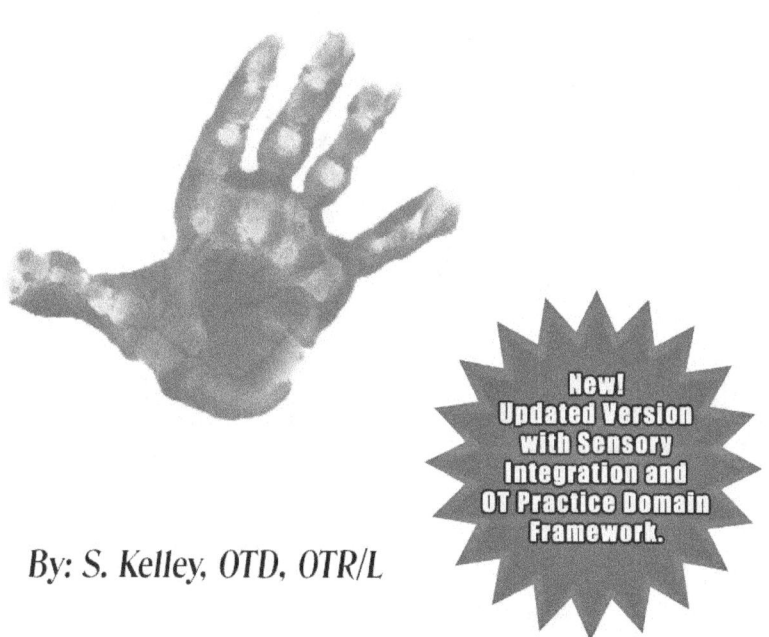

New!
Updated Version with Sensory Integration and OT Practice Domain Framework.

By: S. Kelley, OTD, OTR/L

Purple Toes Books

School Based & Pediatric Occupational Therapy Resource Series:
Quick Pediatric Fine Motor and Sensory Screener & Assessment

S. Kelley

By S Kelley, OTD OTR/L
First Edition
© Purple Toes Books
Http:\\www.purpletoesbooks.com
U.S.A

Dedication

This book is gratefully and gracefully dedicated to all the families and team members that I have shared in my journey.

This is for you.

Acknowledgements

This book and my work as an occupational therapist are made possible by the support and love of many wonderful people. I would like to thank my mentors, colleagues, and team members over the years, over the miles. Each experience has been unique and rewarding and I am thankful to have shared them with you.

I would like to acknowledge my husband for his unwavering support and love. To my parents and grandparents, you have provided me with the foundation for which I have remained grounded.

Special Thanks

To my son. Without your life, love and perseverance I would never know my own strength.

Let Go. Let God.

About the Author

Dr. S. Kelley, OTD, OTR/L currently practices as a pediatric occupational therapist in the school setting. She has facilitated the participation and skill growth for students in both regular education and special education programs. With a background as both an early childhood teacher and occupational therapist, Dr. Kelley has a unique and specialized perspective of education for students. Dr. Kelley specializes in the treatment of students in the early childhood self contained special education classes. After nearly 15 years of practice, Dr. Kelley decided to create resources for the school based and pediatric therapist to help facilitate effective and efficient practice. These resources reflect both the OT Practice Framework (AOTA, 2008) and the Common Core Curriculum (Common Core Standards Initiative, 2012). These resources were then made available in alternative formats for families and parents as a response from families and co-workers.

Dr. Kelley holds a Bachelor of Arts in Early Childhood Education from Clemson University and a Bachelor of Science in Occupational Therapy from University of Wisconsin-Milwaukee. She also holds a Professional Master's and Doctorate degree in Occupational Therapy from Boston University. Dr. Kelley is registered nationally as a specialist in pediatric occupational therapy.

About the *Resource Series* from Purple Toes Books

The purpose of the *Resource Series*, in various formats, is to provide the reader a collection of practice, easy-to-use activities to assist with various motor, language and social skills. The *Resource Series* is a result of over 15 years of practice in pediatric occupational therapy. Over the course of my practice, I have created, developed, borrowed, collaborated, brainstormed, altered and modified countless activities and tasks. I decided to create a written series of my favorite activities as I use them, in the classroom, in the home or in the clinic.

Although I encourage you to read this book and independently apply the activities and/or interventions in your daily practice, classroom or life, please remind yourself that professionals are available to help you if you need advice or direction. These books are designed to be easy-to-use, but various professionals can help with modifications or adaptations if you need them.

Table of Contents

Occupational Therapy in School Setting

Definition of OT in the School Environment

Occupational therapists promote functional activities and engagement of daily routines. Areas of occupation including, but are not limited to: work, play, leisure, social participation, ADL, IADLs and Education. According to IDEA, occupational therapy services in the school setting are a support services for students identified eligible for special education services. Under Part B of IDEA (2004), services are provided through the individual education plan (IEP) to promote academic success and social participation , to access, progress and participation in the educational environment in the least restrictive environment (AOTA, 2012). Under IDEA's Part B (2004) Regulation the Definition of Occupational Therapy includes the following components:

1. Services must be provided by a qualified occupational therapist
2. Services may "improve, develop or restore functions impaired or lost through illness, injury or deprivation"
3. Services may "improve the ability to perform tasks for independent functioning if functions are impaired or lost"
4. Services may "prevent, through early intervention, initial or further impairment or loss of function" (IDEA, 2004)

OT Goals & Outcomes

Through direct, collaborative and consultative services, occupational therapist create individualized goals with focus on outcomes related to:

1. General Classroom Skills/Accessibility/Participation
2. Playground and Sports Accessibility/Participation
3. School Based Self Help Skills
4. Social Participation in the School Setting

5. Mobility in the educational environment
6. Social Emotional Learning
7. Assistive technology in the educational setting
8. Sensory Regulation
9. Pre-vocational and Vocational Needs in the educational setting

Specific Services Occupational Therapists in the School Setting

- Evaluate students' strengths and weaknesses
- Identify modifications to promote participation
- Provide direct interventions to facilitate function and skill acquisition
- Collaborate and consult with teachers and staff regarding student needs to access his/her educational environment

All Student Support Systems

Occupational therapists in the school setting may provide support services for students with and without disability. This is done through early intervening services, including Response to Intervention.

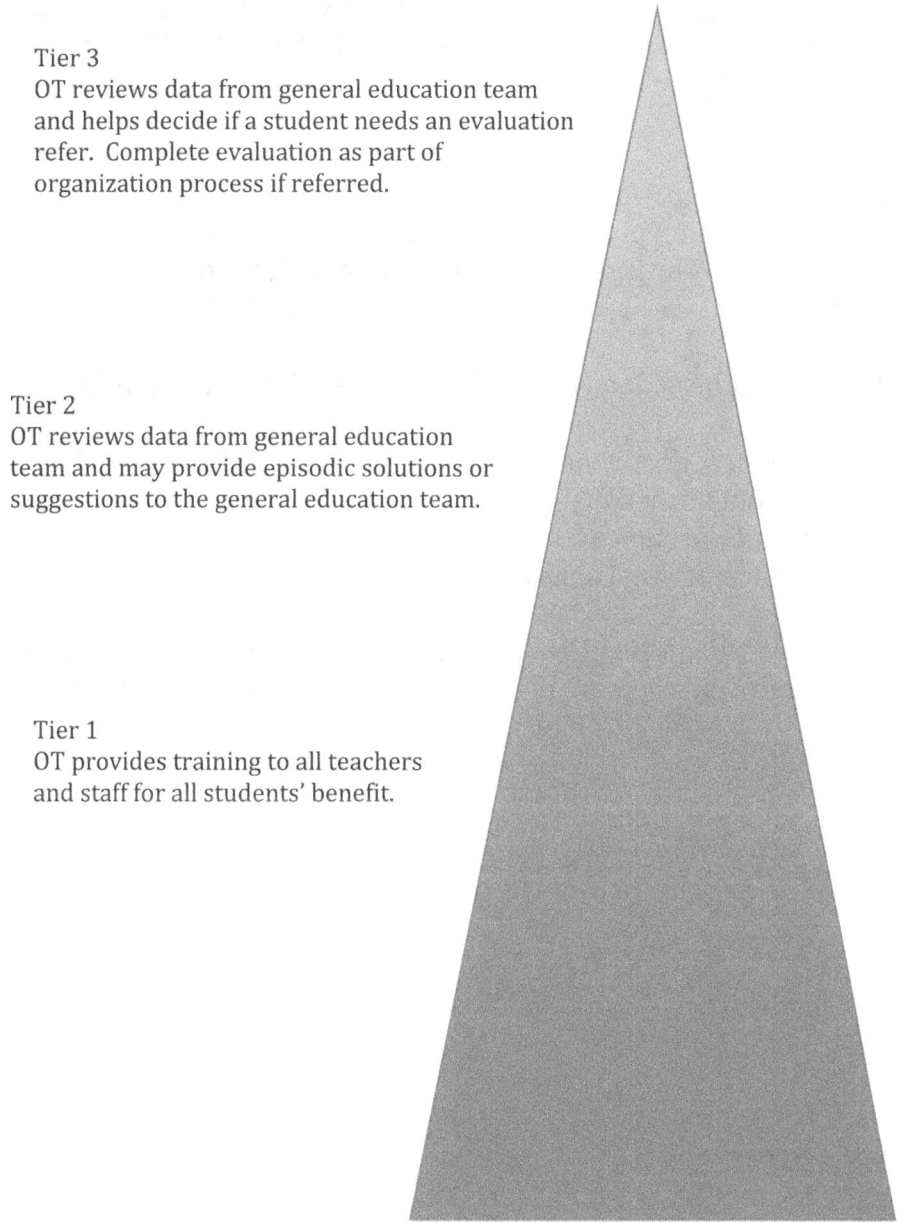

Tier 3
OT reviews data from general education team and helps decide if a student needs an evaluation refer. Complete evaluation as part of organization process if referred.

Tier 2
OT reviews data from general education team and may provide episodic solutions or suggestions to the general education team.

Tier 1
OT provides training to all teachers and staff for all students' benefit.

Resources' Reflection of the OT Practice Framework: Domain and Process (AOTA, 2008).

This book provides a group method to provide services for students with and without disability. Below are the components reflected in the OT Practice Framework (AOTA, 2008) that are potential outcomes of the group treatment.

After the students' occupational profile has been developed, this group serves as the intervention plan, implementation and review within the intervention process. The intervention process includes the following (AOTA, 2008):

- Plan: Guides the actions of the OT and is based on the students' priorities
- Interventions: Carried out actions that address performance skills, patterns, context, activity demands and client factors that are impacting performance
- Review: Allow for revisions in the plan and actions

It should be noted, all interventions have the primary goal to achieving the primary outcome of engagement in occupation to support participation. (AOTA, 2008)

Areas of Occupation

Education
Play
Leisure
Social Participation

Performance Skills

Motor Skills
        Posture (Stabilizes, Aligns, Positions)

Mobility (Walks, Reaches, Bends)
Coordination (Coordinates, Manipulates, Flows)
Strength & Effort (Moves, Transport, Lifts, Calibrates, Grips)
Energy (Endures, Paces)
Process Skills
Energy (Paces, Attends)
Knowledge (Chooses, Uses, Handles, Heeds, Inquires)
Temporal Organization (Initiates, Continues, Sequences, Terminates)
Organizing Space & Objects (Searches, Gathers)

Resources' Connection to the Common Core Curriculum

(National Governors Association Center for Best Practices & Council of Chief State School Officers, 2010).

It is the goal of this assessment to address areas noted in the Common Core Curriculum. Students are asked to rise to the standards and this assessment may help determine areas of weakness or needed development in order to reach these standards.

Below are components connected to the Common Core Curriculum. Due to the nature of the Common Core Domain, only broad standards in Kindergarten are provided. Please see the Common Core Curriculum for additional grades.

English Language Arts

ENGLISH LANGUAGE ARTS STANDARDS: LANGUAGE

CCSS.ELA.Literacy.L.K.1a   Print many upper and lower case letters.

CCSS.ELA.Literacy.L.K.1b   Use frequently occurring nouns and verbs

CCSS.ELA.Literacy.L.K.1c or /es/   Form regular plural nouns orally by adding /s/

CCSS.ELA.Literacy.L.K.1d   Understand and use question words

CCSS.ELA.Literacy.L.K.1e   Use frequently occurring prepositions

CCSS.ELA.Literacy.L.K.1f   Produce and expand complete sentences in shared language

CCSS.ELA.Literacy.L.K.4a   Identify new meanings to new or familiar words

CCSS.ELA.Literacy.L.K.5a   Sort Common objects into categories

CCSS.ELA.Literacy.L.K.6   Use words and phrases acquired through conversations, reading and being read to

ENGLISH LANGUAGE ARTS STANDARDS: SPEAKING AND LISTENING

CCSS.ELA-Literacy.SL.K.1	Participate in collaborative conversations with diverse partners about topics with peers and adults
CCSS.ELA-Literacy.SL.K.1a	Follow rules for discussion (listen to others, taking turns)
CCSS.ELA-Literacy.SL.K.1b	Continue conversation through multiple exchanges
CCSS.ELA-Literacy.SL.K.2	Confirm understanding of text read aloud or information presented orally or through other media by asking and answering questions
CCSS.ELA-Literacy.SL.K.3	Ask and answer questions in order to seek help, get information, or clarify something misunderstood
CCSS.ELA-Literacy.SL.K.4	Describe familiar people, places, things and events with assistance
CCSS.ELA-Literacy.SL.K.5	Add drawings or visuals to provide additional information/details
CCSS.ELA-Literacy.SL.K.6	Speak audibly and express thoughts, feelings, and ideas

ENGLISH LANGUAGE ARTS STANDARDS: READING: FOUNDATIONAL SKILLS

CCSS.ELA.Literacy.RF.K.1a	Follow words from left to right, top to bottom, page to page
CCSS.ELA.Literacy.RF.K.1b	Recognize that spoken words are represented in written form

ENGLISH LANGUAGE ARTS STANDARDS: WRITING

CCSS.ELA.Literacy.W.K.1	Use a combination of drawing, dictating and writing to compose an opinion about the name of a book and preference about it
CCSS.ELA.Literacy.W.K.2	Use a combination of drawing, dictating and writing to create details about a topic
CCSS.ELA.Literacy.W.K.3	Use a combination of drawing, dictating and writing to narrate a single event about a topic
CCSS.ELA.Literacy.W.K.5	With assistance, respond to questions and suggestions to add details and strength writing
CCSS.ELA.Literacy.W.K.6	With assistance, explore a variety of digital tools to produce writing

CCSS.ELA.Literacy.W.K.7	Participate in shared research and writing projects
CCSS.ELA.Literacy.W.K.8	With assistance, recall information from experiences and gather information from sources to answer a question

Mathematics

MATHEMATICS:MEASUREMENT & DATA

CCSS.Math.Content.K.MD.A.1	Describe measurable attributes of objects
CCSS.Math.Content.K.MD.A.2	Directly compare two objects with measurable attributes
CCSS.Math.Content.K.MD.B.3	Classify objects in categories, count, and sort

MATHEMATICS:GEOMETRY

CCSS.Math.Content.K.G.A.1	Describe objects in the environment using names of shapes and use relative positions of these objects (spatial)
CCSS.Math.Content.K.G.A.2	Correctly name shapes
CCSS.Math.Content.K.G.A.3	Identify shapes

MATHEMATICS: COUNTING & CARDINALITY

CCSS.Math.Content.K.CC.A.1	Count to 100 by ones and tens
CCSS.Math.Content.K.CC.B.4	Understand the relationship between numbers and quantities.

Resources' & Sensory Integration Framework
(Ayres, 2005)

Sensory Integration is defined as the organization of sensory input from one's environment and the responses one's body has as a result. It is a complex system that requires the nervous system to work in harmony together to interact with the environment and experiences within it.

Vestibular Response: Sensation from body regarding gravity and movement (knowing where one's head is in space)

Proprioception Response: Sensation from the body, muscles and joints (where the body "feels" itself in space

Tactile/Touch: Feeling through the body, hands, skin

Visual Sense: Seeing what's in space and distinguishing between various visual input

Auditory Sense: Hearing sounds in space and distinguishing between various sound input

Olfactory Sense: Smelling scents in space and distinguishing between various smells

Gustatory Sense: Tasting food in the mouth and distinguishing between different tastes (sour, sweet, etc)

Dysfunctional Response: Negative action or emotional response, lack of response or mismatched response

Fine Motor Assessment & Screener

Use for this Screener

This screener can be used to determine basic skill acquisition, baseline for fine motor skills or to screen for potential need for additional support either through direct therapy services or their Roti support systems.

Grasping Skills

3 years old	Various
3.5 years old	Static Tripod Grasp
4 years old	Dynamic Tripod Grasp Emerging

Prewriting Skills

3 years old	Vertical, Horizontal, Circle
4 years old	Diagonal, Cross, Tracing
5 years old	X, square, triangle, emerging words

Cutting Skills

2 years old	Snip
3 years old	Cut on straight line
4 year old	Cut on straight line, emerging curves
4.5 years old	Cut circles and squares
5 years old	Cut complex shapes, cut without lines

Therapist Data Sheet

Student Name: _____

Classroom: _____

Age: _____

Date of Screener: _____

How is the pencil held?

Radial Cross Palmar Grasp

Palmar Supinate Grasp

Digital Pronate Grasp (3rd extended)

Brush Grasp

Tripod Extended Fingers

Tripod Flexed Fingers

Cross Thumb Grasp

Static Tripod Grasp

Four Finger Grasp

Lateral Tripod Grasp

Tripod Grasp (Functional & Efficient)

Which hand is dominant?

Left   Right   Not Established/Switches

How much pressure is used?

Light   Appropriate   Hard

Can he/she cross midline?   Yes   No

What kind of scissors are used?

Small Loop	Blue Loop	Regular

Is thumb kept up?	Yes	No
Does the helper hand control paper?	Yes	No
Does he/she has independent scissor orientation?	Yes	No

Skills Demonstrated

Imitation Skill Mastered	Date Emerging	Date
Vertical _____	_____	
Horizontal _____	_____	
Circle _____	_____	
Cross _____	_____	

Copying Skill Mastered	Date Emerging	Date
Vertical _____	_____	
Horizontal _____	_____	
Circle _____	_____	
Cross _____	_____	
X _____	_____	
Square _____	_____	

Triangle   _____

Diamond   _____

Draw Person   **Date Emerging**   **Date**
Mastered

Scribble   _____

Head & 2 Arms   _____

Head, More Parts, No Body   _____

4 Body Parts   _____

Add detail with facial   _____

6 Body Parts   _____

Drawing Skill   **Date Emerging**   **Date**
Mastercd

Vertical   _____

Horizontal   _____

Circle   _____

Cross

_____   _____

X

_____   _____

Square

_____   _____

Triangle

_____   _____

Diamond

_____   _____

Coloring in Borders

_____   _____

Handwriting Samples

Skill Mastered	Date Emerging	Date
Trace Name	_____	
Copy Name	_____	
Write Name	_____	

Upper Case   _____

        _____

Lower Case   _____

        _____

Near Pont   _____

        _____

Cutting Samples

Skill Mastered	Date Emerging	Date
Snip	_____	
_____		
Snip Once on Line	_____	
_____		
Consecutive Snipping	_____	
_____		
Cut on Line	_____	
_____		
Cut out Circle	_____	
_____		
Cut out Square	_____	
_____		
Cut out Complex Shape	_____	
_____		
Cut out without Lines	_____	
_____		

Data Collection Sheet

Use this sheet for imitation, copying and drawing. Circle the skill being observed.

IMITATION   COPYING   DRAWING

|	
—	
◯	

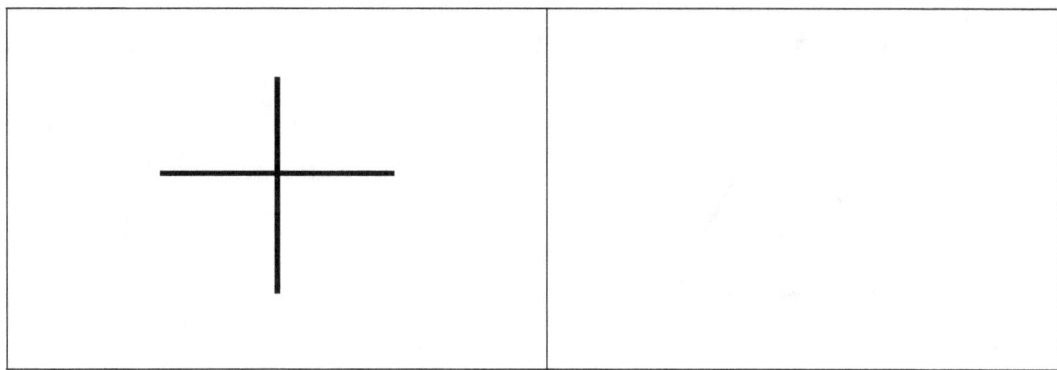

Data Collection Sheet

Use this sheet for imitation, copying and drawing. Circle the skill being observed.

IMITATION   COPYING   DRAWING

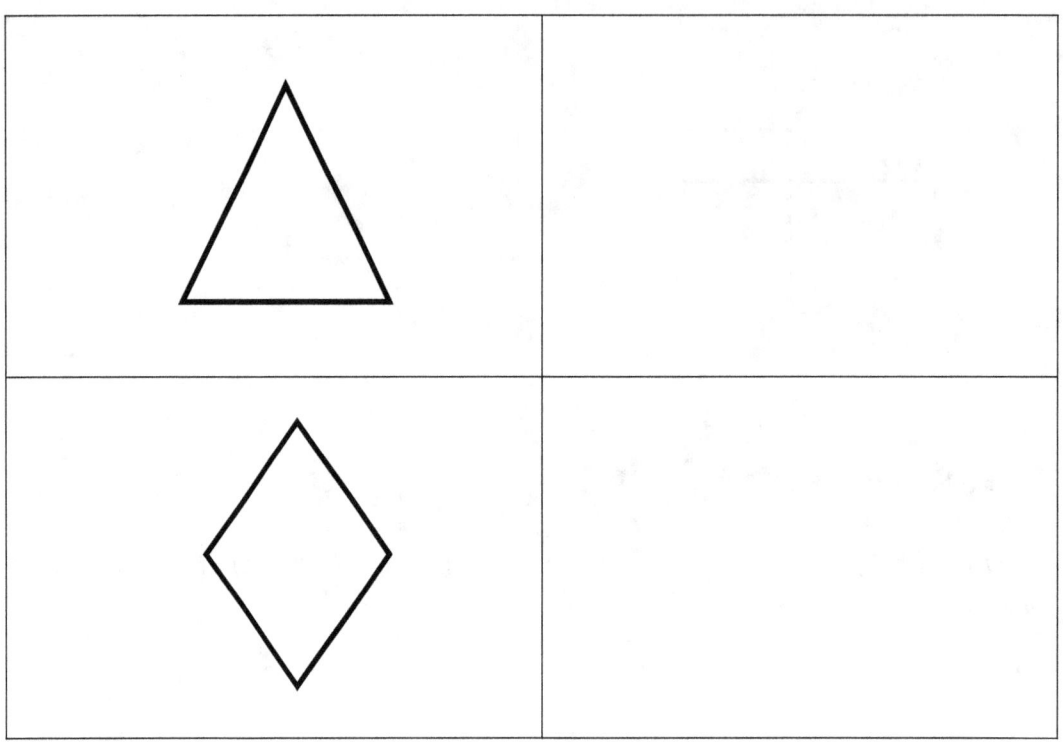

Data Collection

Draw a Person

Count the number of parts drawn.

Data Collection

Coloring

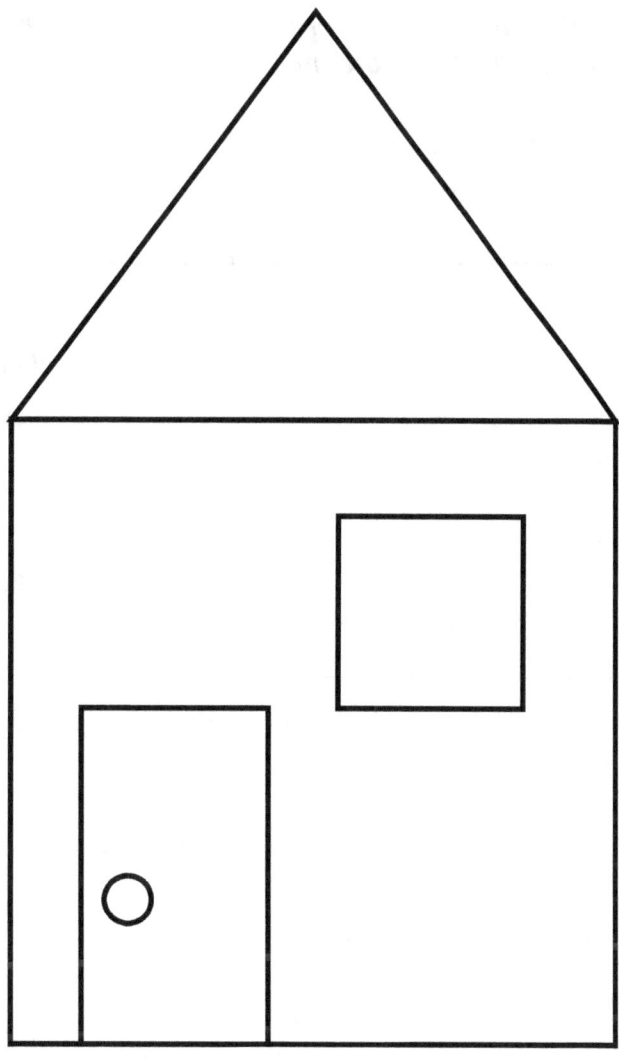

Data Collection

Write student's name in yellow or lined to trace on given line. Determine number of letters legible or attempted.

_____

Write student's name with pencil on line. Have student copy it using near point example.

_____

_____

Ask student to independently write his/her name on the given line.

_____

Data Collection

Write upper case letters on the given line (using your school's desired writing style) Ask student to copy each letter below given example.

_____

_____

_____

_____

_____

_____

_____

_____

Data Collection

Write lower case letters on the given line (using your school's desired writing style) Ask student to copy each letter below given example.

_____

_____

_____

Data Collection

Write simple words on the given line. Ask student to copy each letter below given example.

_____

_____

_____

_____

_____

Data Collection

To collect data on snipping, use a blank sheet or index card.
Precut the line separate from the circle for data collection.

Cut on line

Cut out circle on curved line

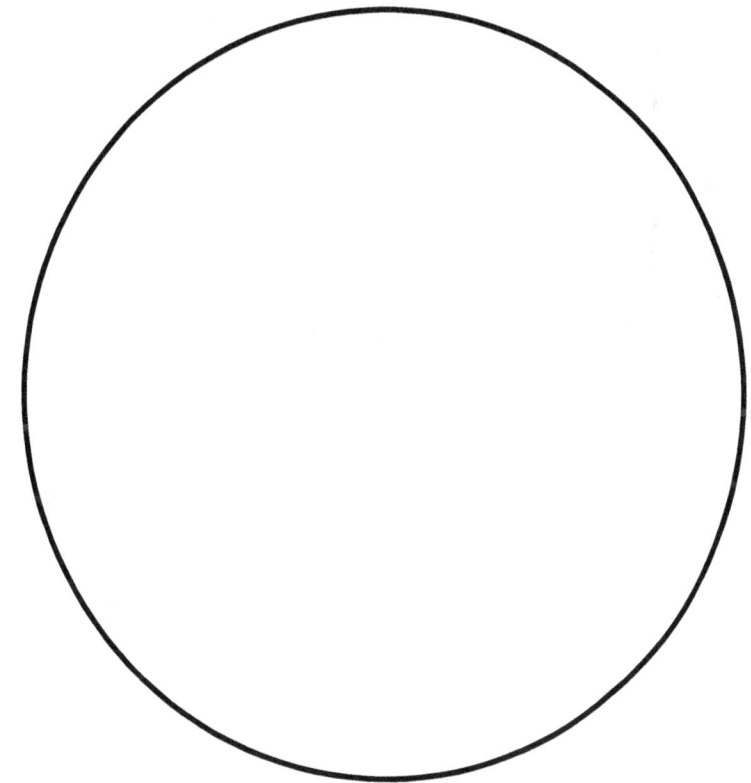

Data Collection

Precut the square separate from the complex shape for data collection.

Cut out square on line

Cut out complex shapes on line

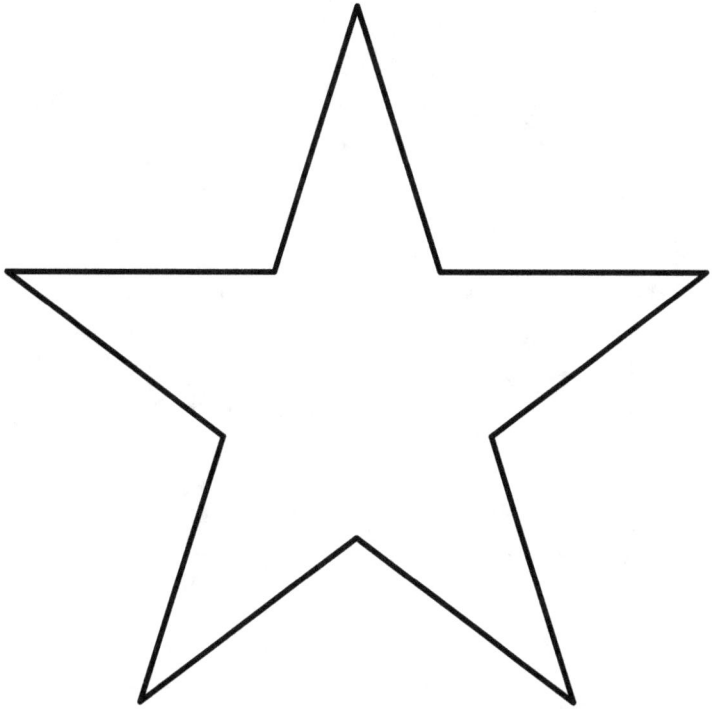

Sensory Screener

Collaborate with team to determine the correct response. "Yes" responses should be highlighted as possible concerns. This may require the need for a formal OT evaluation as well as environmental solutions to promote success in the classroom.

Use this information for screening purposes ONLY

Area of Concern	Yes	No
Hates messy media? Getting hands dirty?		
Moves about the classroom excessively? Can't sit still?		
Struggles to use two hands for tasks? Can't catch a ball, hold a cup		
Uses too much force when coloring or writing? Breaks utensils?		
Struggles to eat a variety of foods? Very picky? Gags with new tastes?		
Puts hands over ears with given auditory input tolerates by peers? Appears distressed?		
Stares at objects? Inconsistent eye contact?		

Inattentiveness to visual detail?		
Restless, fidgety?		
Excessive spinning, bouncing, swinging?		

Results from Sensory Screener

Sensory System Correlated to Question	Concern?
Tactile Defensiveness	
Sensory Seeker/Vestibular/Proprioceptive	
Bilateral Integration Function	
Proprioception	
Tactile Defensiveness/Oral Defensiveness	
Auditory Defensiveness	
Visual Sensory Needs	
Sensory Seeking/Vestibular/Proprioceptive	
Sensory Seeking/Vestibular/Proprioceptive	

Informal Observations/Concerns

References

American Occupational Therapy Association. (2008). Occupational therapy practice framework: Domain and process (2nd ed.). American Journal of Occupational Therapy , 62, 625–683.

American Occupational Therapy Association (2012). Role of Occupational Therapy with Children and Youth with Children and Youth in School in School-Based Practice.

Ayres, A. J. (2005). *Sensory integration and the child: 25th anniversary edition.* Lost Angeles, CA: Western Psychological Services.

Individuals With Disabilities Education Act, 20 U.S.C. § 1400 (2004).

National Governors Association Center for Best Practices & Council of Chief State School Officers. (2010). *Common Core State Standards.* Washington, DC: Authors.

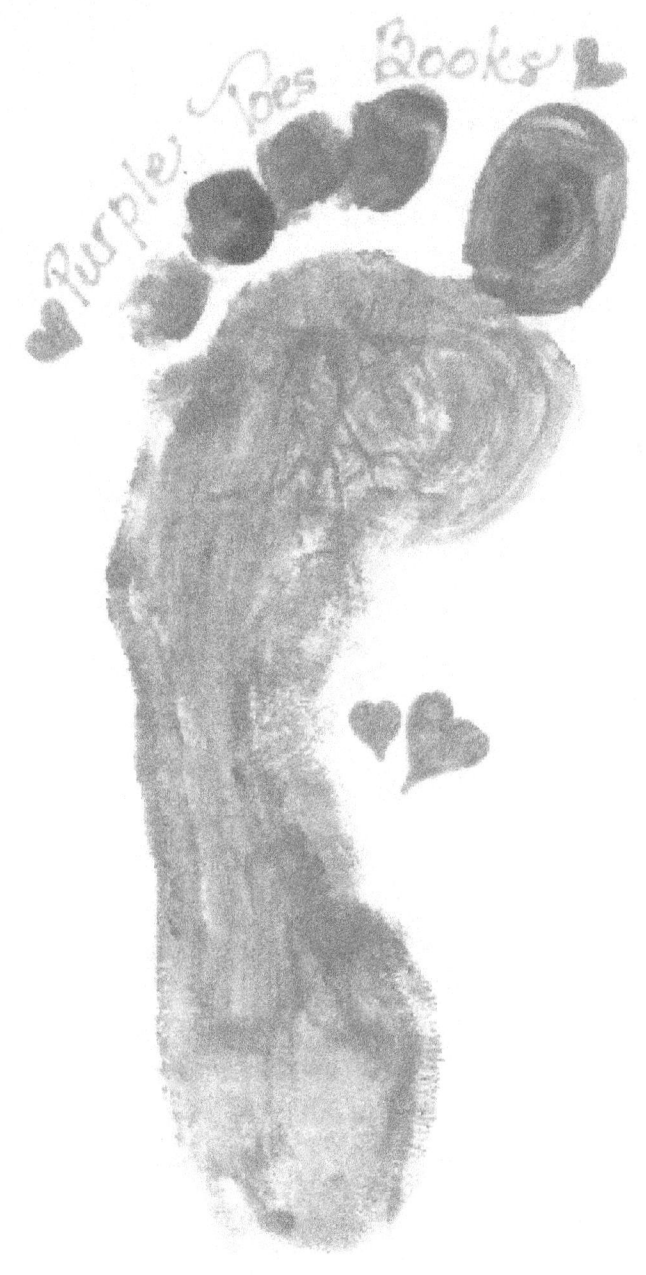

Purple Toes Books